KNOWLEDGE GUIDE TO OSGOOD SCHLATTER DISEASE

Essential Manual To Causes, Symptoms, Diagnosis, Treatment, And Pain Management For Active Adolescents And Athletes

DR. AARON BRANUM

Copyright © 2024 BY DR. AARON BRANUM

All rights reserved. Except for brief quotations embodied in critical reviews and certain other noncommercial uses permitted by copyright law, no part of this publication may be reproduced, distributed, or transmitted in any form or by any means, Including photocopying, recording, or other electronic or mechanical methods, without the prior written permission of the publisher.

Disclaimer:

The data in this book, is solely meant to be informative and instructional.

This book is not intended to replace expert medical advice, diagnosis, or care. No medical, health, or other professional services are offered by the author, publisher, or any affiliated parties

Individual outcomes may differ in the practice of these therapies, which entail a variety of approaches and methodologies.

A one-on-one session with a trained or certified healthcare professional is still preferable. It is best to consult a trained healthcare provider before making any decisions regarding your health.

The author of this book is not affiliated with any specific website, product, or organization related to any of these therapies.

All reasonable measures have been taken by the author and publisher to guarantee the authenticity and dependability of the material contained in this book

Contents

CHAPTER ONE 13
GAINING INSIGHT INTO OSGOOD SCHLATTER DISEASE 13
Background And Definition 13
Reasons And Danger Elements 14
Growth Spurts And Their Function 15
Physiology Of The Affected Region 16

CHAPTER TWO 21
INDICATES AND SYMPTOMS 21
Description And Location Of The Pain 21
Adrenalization And Inflammation 22
Variations In Levels Of Physical Activity ... 23
Effects On Daily Life And Athletic Engagement 24
Symptoms' Development Over Time 25

CHAPTER THREE 27
DIAGNOSIS PROCEDURE 27
Clinical Assessment By A Medical Professional 27
Methods Of Physical Examination 28

Using Imaging Studies (Mris And X-Rays).30
A Look At Differential Diagnosis 31
The Value Of Interaction With The Medical Staff 33
CHAPTER FOUR 35
OPTIONS FOR TREATMENT 35
Rest And Adjusting Activities 35
Techniques For Pain Management...........36
Exercises For Physical Therapy................37
Devices For Bracing And Supporting 38
Surgical Procedures (Very Rare)..............38
CHAPTER FIVE 41
MEASURES TO PREVENT OSGOOD-SCHLATTER DISEASE..............................41
The Value Of Warming Up And Cooling Down 41
Appropriate Form And Technique In Sports 43
Progressive Intensification And Lengthening Of Activities 44
Instruction On Injury Prevention Techniques 46

CHAPTER SIX 49
MANAGEMENT METHODS 49
The Disease's Psychological Effects 51
Systems Of Support For Patients And Their Families 53
Recovering With Reasonable Expectations 55
Modifications To Lifestyle And Activities 57
Campaigns For Awareness And Advocacy . 60

CHAPTER SEVEN 63
RECTIFICATION METHOD 63
Gradual Resumption Of Physical Activity ... 63
Sports Medicine Specialists And Physical Therapists' Roles 64
Extended-Term Management Approaches . 66

CHAPTER EIGHT 67
LIFESTYLE MODIFICATIONS 67
Nutritional Aspects Of Healing And Recuperation 67
Ergonomic Modifications For Everyday Tasks 68
Including Low-Impact Activities 70

6

The Value Of Getting Enough Sleep And Rest 71
Taking Rest Periods And Physical Activity Into Account 72
CHAPTER NINE 75
RESEARCH DIRECTIONS AND FUTURE STEPS 75
New Approaches To Treatment 75
Progress In Diagnostic Methods 77
Knowing The Long-Term Prognosis 80

CONCERNING THIS BOOK

The "Knowledge Guide to Osgood Schlatter Disease" is an invaluable tool for anyone looking for in-depth information on this common knee illness, which primarily affects teenagers.

The definition and history of Osgood Schlatter Disease are thoroughly explored in the book, which lays a solid foundation for readers' comprehension of the condition's causes, risk factors, and the crucial role growth spurts play in its development. Understanding this background is essential to understanding how the affected area's anatomy is specifically harmed, setting it apart from other knee ailments.

A detailed examination of Osgood Schlatter Disease's symptoms is provided in the section on signs and symptoms, which highlights the precise pain descriptions, locations, and related swelling and inflammation. Readers must comprehend the significance of early indicators and how alterations in physical activity levels can impact the advancement of symptoms. The disease's wider effects on a person's routine and athletic involvement are highlighted by a thorough examination of the influence on everyday life and sports participation.

The in-depth coverage of diagnosis leads readers through the process of clinical evaluation by medical professionals. The book goes into detail on how to conduct a physical examination and how to properly diagnose a condition using imaging tests like MRIs and X-rays. A correct diagnosis is essential due to its complexity, which is further highlighted by the significance of differential diagnosis considerations and good communication with the healthcare team.

The book discusses treatment choices in detail, including everything from physical therapy exercises and pain management to rest and activity moderation. There is a discussion of the function of bracing and supportive devices, with the observation that surgery is only seldom required. Additionally, preventive measures are highlighted, supporting the value of appropriate sports techniques, gradual increases in exercise intensity, and warm-up and cool-down procedures. This part emphasizes the importance of a balanced approach to physical activity while educating readers on injury avoidance.

In addition, the book explores coping mechanisms, recognizing the psychological effects of the illness on both patients and their families. It provides direction on creating support networks, establishing reasonable goals for recovery, and implementing the required lifestyle changes. Emphasis is placed on advocacy and awareness campaigns, which promote a feeling of solidarity and support.

The value of rehabilitation is emphasized, along with the necessity of tracking progress and symptoms. Rehabilitation is described as a gradual return to physical activities. The significance of physical therapists and sports medicine experts is emphasized, in addition to the incorporation of strengthening and conditioning regimens for extended care. To enhance general healing and well-being, lifestyle adaptations are advised, such as dietary considerations, ergonomic adjustments, and the inclusion of low-impact workouts.

The book discusses new treatment modalities and improvements in diagnostic methods as it looks to the future.

It provides insight into the long-term prognosis of Osgood Schlatter's Disease and emphasizes international initiatives to increase awareness. The possibilities for patient participation in research are outlined, enticing readers to take an active role in the ongoing investigation of this illness.

CHAPTER ONE

GAINING INSIGHT INTO OSGOOD SCHLATTER DISEASE

Background And Definition

For developing teenagers, Osgood Schlatter disease (OSD) is a prevalent cause of knee pain.

The patellar tendon's attachment to the tibia, directly below the knee, is characterized by inflammation in this region.

During growth spurts, when bones, muscles, tendons, and other structures are quickly altering, this syndrome frequently manifests.

It usually affects kids between the ages of 10 and 15 who play sports that require them to run, leap, or change direction quickly.

Recognizing the relationship between development, exercise, and the body's reaction to physical stress during growth is essential to understanding OSD.

Reasons And Danger Elements

Repetitive strain and stress on the growth plate at the top of the shinbone (tibia) are the main causes of Osgood-Schlatter disease.

Running and jumping are two exercises that cause the quadriceps muscle to strain on the patellar tendon, causing tension. Among the risk factors are:

Age and Growth Spurts: Between the ages of 10 and 15, when growth is most rapid, OSD is most common.

Activity Level: Playing sports like basketball, gymnastics, and soccer that require a lot of sprinting, jumping, and sudden direction changes.

Gender: Although OSD can affect males and girls equally, it affects boys more frequently. However, as more females get involved in sports, the gender gap is decreasing.

Genetics: The chance of having OSD may rise if there is a family history of the disorder.

Growth Spurts And Their Function

Growth spurts have a major role in the emergence of OSD. Bones grow quickly during these times, and the muscles and tendons may tense up trying to keep up with the changes.

Tension on the patellar tendon attachment site may increase as a result of the muscles and tendons being comparatively shorter and tighter due to the fast skeletal growth.

Tension like this might cause inflammation and microtrauma at the bony protrusion below the knee called the tibial tuberosity.

The pain and edema that are typical of OSD are caused by the body's attempt to heal this tiny injury.

Physiology Of The Affected Region

The following are the main anatomical structures implicated in Osgood Schlatter disease:

The patellar tendon is the tendon that joins the tibia (the shinbone) to the kneecap (patella). It is essential for knee extension and impact absorption during activity.

The bony protrusion below the kneecap on which the patellar tendon is attached is known as the tibial tuberosity.

This area becomes painfully inflamed when someone has OSD.

Growth Plate (Epiphyseal Plate): A layer of cartilage located in children's and adolescents' long bone ends. As the site of bone formation, it is vulnerable to damage and inflammation during periods of rapid growth.

Knowing the anatomy makes it easier to understand why OSD mostly affects adolescents during growth spurts and why it causes localized discomfort and edema.

Recognizing Osgood Schlatter Differentially from Other Knee Conditions

Osgood Schlatter's disease can be distinguished from other knee problems by taking into account the age range that is affected as well as the particular symptoms. Typical circumstances to set yourself apart from include:

Patellar Tendinitis: This condition, which is more common in adults, is an inflammation of the patellar tendon itself as opposed to OSD, which affects the growth plate.

Jumper's Knee: This condition affects the patellar tendon as well, but it starts at the point where the tendon attaches to the kneecap as opposed to the tibia.

Patellofemoral Pain Syndrome: Unlike OSD, which is characterized by localized discomfort around the tibial tuberosity, this ailment usually manifests as diffuse knee pain around the kneecap.

Meniscal Injuries: These are injuries to the knee's cartilage that frequently cause locking or clicking in the knee, which is not a sign of OSD.

A thorough diagnosis frequently combines a patient's medical history, a physical examination, and occasionally imaging tests like X-rays to rule out other illnesses and establish the existence of alterations in the tibial tuberosity.

CHAPTER TWO

INDICATES AND SYMPTOMS

Description And Location Of The Pain

The primary symptom of Osgood-Schlatter disease is localized pain in the tibial tuberosity, the bony protuberance located directly below the knee cap.

Activities that strain the knee, such as jogging, leaping, and stair climbing, usually make this pain worse.

One's capacity to perform physical tasks may be negatively impacted by pain that ranges from moderate discomfort to severe, incapacitating agony.

Teenagers experiencing discomfort may characterize it as an uncomfortable or sharp sensation that gets better with movement and becomes better with rest. Up to 30% of occurrences of this soreness are bilateral, meaning that while it can be more severe in one knee, it is typically bilateral.

Adrenalization And Inflammation

One of the most prevalent symptoms of Osgood-Schlatter disease is swelling in addition to discomfort.

The tibial tuberosity might be enlarged and swollen to a noticeable extent. The patellar tendon's inflammation at the point where it joins to the tibial tuberosity is the cause of this swelling.

In addition, the region can be warm and sensitive to the touch, suggesting continued inflammation.

A solid, bony lump may occasionally emerge as new bone grows in reaction to the stress.

This lump may remain long after the swelling and agony have decreased, forming an enduring physical feature of the illness.

Variations In Levels Of Physical Activity

Osgood-Schlatter disease frequently causes notable changes in the amount of physical activity that children and teenagers engage in. Sports and other physical activities may see a decline in involvement as a result of the pain and discomfort.

Running, jumping, and kneeling are some of the more difficult activities to perform. Consequently, those who are impacted may participate in fewer sporting events, games, and physical education sessions.

For young athletes who are keen to play their favorite activities but are limited by the disease's pain, this decrease in activity can be upsetting.

Effects On Daily Life And Athletic Engagement

Osgood-Schlatter disease can have a significant effect on day-to-day activities, especially for adolescents who lead busy lives.

The continuous discomfort and swelling can impede regular tasks such as walking, climbing stairs, and even sitting for extended periods with the knee bent.

Participation in sports is frequently severely impacted; many young athletes are forced to reduce or stop playing competitive sports for a while.

Feelings of frustration, loneliness, and worry may result from this, especially if the person's identity is strongly connected to their athletic achievement.

Parents and coaches need to support these youngsters by encouraging relaxation and providing alternative activities that do not increase the symptoms.

Symptoms' Development Over Time

The symptoms of Osgood-Schlatter disease might progress differently in each individual. At first, the discomfort may come on suddenly, just after engaging in vigorous physical activity, and go away when you relax.

With less strenuous activities or even during moments of relaxation, the pain may become more chronic as the illness worsens.

Over time, the soreness and swelling could get worse. Sometimes the symptoms continue for months or even years, but they usually go away by the time adolescence ends and the growth plates close.

But the length and severity of the symptoms might differ greatly, with some people suffering for a long time and others getting better rather rapidly.

CHAPTER THREE

DIAGNOSIS PROCEDURE

Clinical Assessment By A Medical Professional

Usually, an orthopedic specialist or primary care physician, a thorough clinical evaluation is the first step in diagnosing Osgood-Schlatter Disease (OSD).

To fully understand the patient's symptoms, their development, and any behaviors that can exacerbate them, a thorough medical history is taken before beginning this evaluation.

The patient's physical activity level will be questioned by the healthcare professional, especially if they play activities that require sprinting, jumping, or kneeling.

An accurate diagnosis depends on being able to pinpoint a pattern and timeframe for the symptoms, which is made possible by this thorough history.

The patient's growth history will also be evaluated by the physician since OSD frequently manifests during adolescent growth spurts.

It is also critical to comprehend the patient's general health as well as any prior knee ailments or traumas that may have affected the current symptoms.

Setting the stage for the subsequent stages of the diagnostic procedure is this comprehensive clinical evaluation.

Methods Of Physical Examination

The medical professional will concentrate on the knee region during the physical examination, searching for particular indications of OSD. Visual examination of the knee will be performed to check for symptoms such as edema, redness, or odd lumps below the kneecap, which are indicative of the disorder.

A common diagnostic procedure for OSD is palpation, which involves lightly pushing on the knee and the region surrounding the tibial tuberosity to find painful spots and confirm the existence of discomfort.

Along with evaluating the knee joint's range of motion, the medical professional will look for any restrictions or pain when moving the knee.

This entails instructing the patient to execute particular motions, like squatting, jumping, flexing, and extending the knee.

To distinguish OSD from other possible causes of knee discomfort, it is helpful to watch how these movements impact the patient's knee.

Confirming the initial suspicion of OSD based on the clinical evaluation is mostly dependent on the physical examination.

Using Imaging Studies (Mris And X-Rays)

Imaging investigations are frequently used by healthcare providers to support the diagnosis of OSD. The most popular imaging method for OSD diagnosis is X-rays.

They can show distinctive ossification or fragmentation alterations in the tibial tuberosity.

A clear image of the bone structure and any anomalies that support the diagnosis can be obtained with X-rays.

In certain situations, an MRI (Magnetic Resonance Imaging) may be performed, especially if the diagnosis is unclear or if there are unusual symptoms.

An MRI provides a more thorough image of the muscles, tendons, and cartilage surrounding the knee.

It can assist in ruling out other illnesses like tendinitis or a fracture that could resemble the symptoms of OSD.

Imaging investigations offer a thorough view of soft tissue in addition to bone, making them useful tools for confirming OSD.

A Look At Differential Diagnosis

To guarantee the right course of treatment, it is essential to distinguish OSD from other possible knee disorders.

The medical professional has to rule out fractures, juvenile rheumatoid arthritis, and patellar tendinitis as additional causes of knee discomfort in teenagers. Accurate classification is crucial because each of these illnesses has unique characteristics and treatment regimens.

For instance, patellar tendinitis, which might mimic OSD symptoms, usually entails discomfort in the tendon that connects the kneecap to the shinbone.

Conversely, juvenile rheumatoid arthritis typically affects many joints and is associated with systemic symptoms such as weariness and fever, but it can also cause joint pain and swelling.

Knowing these differential diagnoses guarantees that the medical professional can confidently establish OSD and rule out other diseases.

The Value Of Interaction With The Medical Staff

Throughout the diagnostic procedure, good communication between the patient, their family, and the medical staff is essential. Accurate reporting of all symptoms and a thorough understanding of the patient's history are ensured via clear communication.

It also enables the medical professional to inform the patient's family about the diagnosis, available therapies, and the anticipated course of the illness.

Maintaining an open channel of communication guarantees that the patient receives complete treatment and helps to manage expectations.

Monitor the condition and modify therapies as needed, it also promotes adherence to treatment programs and follow-up sessions.

With the assistance of primary care physicians, orthopedic specialists, and potentially physical therapists, the patient can effectively navigate the diagnosis and management of OSD thanks to the collaborative approach of the healthcare team.

CHAPTER FOUR

OPTIONS FOR TREATMENT

Rest And Adjusting Activities

The two most important initial stages in addressing Osgood-Schlatter disease are rest and activity moderation.

This strategy mainly entails cutting back on or giving up on activities like running, jumping, and other high-impact sports that aggravate knee discomfort.

 Alternatively, to maintain general fitness without overstressing the affected area, low-impact exercises like cycling or swimming might be encouraged.

Sufficient rest intervals are necessary to promote healing of the inflamed tissue. A well-balanced routine that alternates between work and relaxation can greatly reduce symptoms and stop them from getting worse.

Techniques For Pain Management

For Osgood-Schlatter disease patients to receive relief and have a higher quality of life, pain management is essential.

Acetaminophen or ibuprofen are examples of over-the-counter drugs that can help lower pain and inflammation.

Another way to reduce swelling and numb the pain in the knee is to apply ice packs many times a day for 15 to 20 minutes each time.

When at rest, elevating the leg can help minimize swelling even more. Heat pads can also help release tight muscles surrounding the knee before exercises.

Exercises For Physical Therapy

Osgood-Schlatter disease symptoms can be lessened with the use of physical therapy exercises, which help strengthen the knee muscles and increase flexibility.

Exercises that stretch the hamstrings and quadriceps can ease the strain on the patellar tendon.

Supportive muscle strength can be increased with strengthening activities such as leg presses, hamstring curls, and calf lifts. Exercises for balance and coordination help enhance knee stability overall.

A physical therapist can create an exercise program specifically tailored to each patient's needs and make sure activities are done correctly to prevent the recurrence of injury.

Devices For Bracing And Supporting

Supportive equipment and bracing provide the knee with more stability and less strain. During athletic exercises, knee braces or straps—like patellar tendon straps—can be worn to support the knee and deflect stress away from the irritated area.

These gadgets might lessen discomfort when moving and provide users the confidence to partake in mild activities without making their condition worse. Maximum benefit and comfort are ensured with proper fitting and usage instructions from a healthcare practitioner.

Surgical Procedures (Very Rare)

For Osgood-Schlatter disease, surgery is rarely necessary and is only used as a last resort. When non-invasive therapies have proven ineffective and the pain keeps coming back or gets worse, severely impairing everyday functioning, surgery may be considered. To relieve pressure and pain, the inflammatory tissue or bone overgrowth is usually removed during the surgery.

A well-designed rehabilitation program is essential to regaining knee strength and function after surgery.

Surgery is only advised when required and following a complete evaluation by an orthopedic specialist due to the invasiveness and hazards involved.

CHAPTER FIVE

MEASURES TO PREVENT OSGOOD-SCHLATTER DISEASE

Osgood-Schlatter disease (OSD) is a prevalent ailment among adolescents who lead active lives, especially those involved in sports. Implementing preventive actions can help lower the risk and severity of OSD, even though it frequently resolves on its own.

The Value Of Warming Up And Cooling Down

The body is better prepared for the demands of exercise when it warms up before playing sports or doing other physical activities. A good warm-up improves joint mobility, increases blood flow to the muscles, and increases muscle flexibility. This can be accomplished by engaging in mild cardiovascular activities like cycling or jogging, and then stretching your quadriceps, hamstrings, and calves dynamically.

By preparing the knee-supporting muscles and tendons for the subsequent, more strenuous exercise, these activities may lessen the load on the tibial tuberosity.

Likewise, it's important to cool down after working out. By progressively lowering heart rate and aiding in the removal of lactic acid accumulation in the muscles, this procedure helps avoid stiffness and pain.

Gentle cardiovascular exercise and static stretching that concentrates on the muscles used during the activity should be part of the cooling down process.

This exercise aids in preserving muscle elasticity and guards against injuries, such as OSD.

Appropriate Form And Technique In Sports

Preventing injuries during sports and physical activities requires maintaining good form and technique. Trainers and coaches need to stress proper biomechanics during exercises like jumping, jogging, and landing. One way to assist in distributing pressures equally across the knee joint and lessen stress on the patellar tendon is for an athlete to land with their knees slightly bent and aligned with their toes.

Athletes can form positive habits by receiving corrective feedback and routine technique evaluations. Another important factor is to choose equipment that promotes good form, such as shoes with sufficient cushioning and support. In addition to improving performance, appropriate technique reduces the chance of acquiring disorders such as OSD.

Progressive Intensification And Lengthening Of Activities

Overuse injuries such as OSD can result from abrupt increases in the volume, duration, or intensity of physical activity, beyond the body's capacity for adaptation.

A training program's advancement must be made gradually. As their strength and endurance increase, athletes should progressively increase the intensity and duration of their workouts.

By taking small steps, the body can gradually strengthen its bones, muscles, and tendons in response to increasing demands. Training regimens should include rest days to allow the body to heal and rebuild.

It can also be helpful to alter training loads appropriately to prevent injuries by keeping an eye out for indicators of overuse, such as chronic soreness or swelling.

Including Exercises for Strengthening and Stretching

Exercises that combine stretching and strengthening are essential for preventing OSD. Enhancing the strength of the knee-supporting muscles, specifically the hamstrings, calf, and quadriceps, aids in stabilizing the knee joint and reducing impact during exercise.

The required muscle strength can be developed with exercises including lunges, squats, leg presses, and calf lifts.

Frequent stretching exercises are necessary to preserve joint range of motion and muscle flexibility in addition to strengthening.

Reducing muscular stress and tightness around the knee can be achieved by stretching the quadriceps, hamstrings, and calves. Strength and flexibility training can be seamlessly incorporated into a regular program with the help of yoga and pilates.

Instruction On Injury Prevention Techniques

Parents, coaches, and athletes must receive education on preventing injuries. It can be easier to identify and treat OSD early on if one is aware of the risk factors, symptoms, and preventative techniques.

Workshops, instruction, and educational resources can impart important knowledge on how to safeguard the knees and general musculoskeletal health.

It is important to teach athletes to pay attention to their bodies and to report any pain or discomfort as soon as they feel it.

Trainers and coaches can design training regimens with steady advancement and rest intervals, teach proper warm-up and cool-down procedures, and model good form and technique.

A culture of preventive and awareness-raising can greatly lower the frequency of overuse injuries, including OSD.

CHAPTER SIX

MANAGEMENT METHODS

Osgood-Schlatter disease can be difficult to manage, particularly for young athletes who have a strong love for their activities. Nonetheless, several techniques can be used to control the illness's symptoms and lessen its interference with day-to-day activities.

First of all, it's critical to pay attention to your body and refrain from overexerting oneself. To allow the pain and inflammation to go down, rest is essential. This could entail abstaining from high-impact sports or other activities until the symptoms subside. It's also critical to let coaches, instructors, and parents know about your illness so they can support you and make the appropriate modifications.

Adding low-impact workouts to your regimen can also help you stay active without aggravating your symptoms. Exercises that are less taxing on the knees but effective include swimming, cycling, and yoga. Exercises for strengthening the quadriceps, hamstrings, and calves can also aid with knee joint stabilization and lessen patellar tendon tension.

Furthermore, employing pain management methods like knee braces, cold packs, and over-the-counter painkillers can offer momentary alleviation from discomfort. Enhancing knee proprioception, strength, and flexibility may also be advantageous with physical therapy.

Coping with Osgood-Schlatter's disease can be greatly improved by keeping a positive outlook and asking for help from friends, family, and medical experts. Keep in mind that the illness is typically just momentary, and most people may resume their regular activities without any long-term effects if they receive the right care.

The Disease's Psychological Effects

Osgood-Schlatter disease can have a substantial psychological impact in addition to its physical effects, particularly in young athletes who have a strong passion for their activity. Feelings of irritation, worry, and even melancholy can arise from managing chronic pain, limits in one's activities, and the dread of not being able to function as well as one once could.

Osgood-Schlatter disease sufferers must recognize and deal with these emotional difficulties. Asking for help from friends, family, coaches, and medical professionals can be a great way to let your emotions out and get support. Joining online forums or support groups where people discuss their experiences with the illness can also help foster a sense of community and lessen feelings of loneliness.

Using stress-reduction methods like mindfulness, deep breathing, and meditation can also assist manage the disease's psychological effects. These methods can raise mood, encourage relaxation, and improve general well-being.

In addition, despite the limits imposed by Osgood-Schlatter disease, people can preserve a feeling of identity and purpose by concentrating on parts of life outside of sports. Outside of sporting interests, pursuing hobbies, spending time with loved ones, and achieving academic or professional goals can all lead to a sense of pleasure and success.

In general, treating the psychological effects of Osgood-Schlatter disease is a crucial part of providing complete care for those who have this illness. Through identification and proactive handling of the psychological obstacles linked to the illness, people can enhance their general quality of life and overall state of health.

Systems Of Support For Patients And Their Families

Osgood-Schlatter disease can be extremely difficult to manage, both for the afflicted person and their family. Coping with the obstacles the disease presents can be greatly aided by having a solid support system in place.

Support for patients can come from a variety of people, such as friends, coaches, instructors, and medical professionals. People who have Osgood-Schlatter disease must be transparent with their support system about their needs, worries, and limitations. This can guarantee that they have the support, understanding, and encouragement they need to manage the illness well.

Families of those who suffer from Osgood-Schlatter disease are also essential sources of encouragement and support. This could be assisting with everyday tasks, driving patients to appointments, and providing emotional support through trying times. Family members must be knowledgeable about the illness to better comprehend its effects and know how to care for their loved ones.

Community resources are available to assist individuals and families impacted by Osgood-Schlatter disease, in addition to personal support networks. Support groups, internet discussion boards, and instructional resources offered by advocacy and healthcare groups are a few examples of this.

Strong support networks help Osgood-Schlatter disease sufferers and their families better manage the difficulties the illness presents and enhance their general quality of life.

Recovering With Reasonable Expectations

Osgood-Schlatter disease recovery necessitates tolerance, perseverance, and reasonable expectations. It's crucial to realize that mending takes time and that pushing too hard might worsen symptoms and postpone recovery, even if the condition can be unpleasant and restricting at times.

Accepting the constraints imposed by the disease and emphasizing steady development rather than expecting instant outcomes are key components of setting realistic expectations. To enable the body to heal appropriately, this can entail temporarily cutting back on or altering sports and other high-impact activities.

It's also critical to heed medical professionals' advice and stick to prescribed treatment regimens.

This could involve changing activities, ice therapy, physical therapy, pain management strategies, and rest. Recovery and the likelihood of problems are facilitated and reduced when patients adhere to treatment suggestions consistently.

Furthermore, it's critical to pay attention to your body and avoid pushing past discomfort. Ignoring pain might make the illness worse and make recovery take longer. Rather, observe how your body reacts to various tasks and make necessary adjustments to prevent aggravating symptoms.

Ultimately, staying motivated during the healing process can be achieved by keeping an optimistic outlook and concentrating on minor victories along the road.

Honor the efforts made toward healing and celebrate any improvement, no matter how tiny.

Osgood-Schlatter disease patients can maximize their chances of a successful outcome by establishing reasonable expectations and approaching recovery with patience and determination.

Modifications To Lifestyle And Activities

Adapting one's lifestyle and hobbies to the constraints imposed by Osgood-Schlatter's disease may be necessary when living with the condition. While this might be tough, various ways can help patients retain a full and active lifestyle while limiting the impact of the disease.

Firstly, it's necessary to emphasize activities that are soft on the knees and avoid those that increase symptoms.

This may mean altering sports or finding alternative forms of exercise that place less stress on the patellar tendon.

Low-impact activities such as swimming, cycling, and yoga might give excellent alternatives that allow folks to keep active without aggravating their symptoms.

Additionally, including strength and flexibility exercises in the daily routine can assist improve knee stability and lower the chance of injury.

To increase the strength and stability surrounding the knee joint, concentrate on workouts that work the hamstrings, quadriceps, and calf muscles.

Furthermore, minimizing knee strain and lowering the likelihood of flare-ups can be achieved by paying attention to good body mechanics and posture during exercises.

Repetitive leaping or squatting exercises should be avoided since they may aggravate Osgood-Schlatter disease symptoms.

Ultimately, leading a healthy lifestyle that incorporates appropriate eating, drinking, and sleeping patterns can promote general physical well-being and speed Osgood-Schlatter disease recovery.

People can manage their symptoms and continue to lead active, satisfying lives by mindfully modifying their lifestyles and activities.

Campaigns For Awareness And Advocacy

Enhancing knowledge, resources, and support for those impacted by Osgood-Schlatter disease is mostly dependent on advocacy and awareness campaigns.

Osgood-Schlatter disease patients can live better lives thanks to the efforts of individuals and groups that advocate for improved treatment options and support services as well as increase public knowledge of the condition.

Educating the public on Osgood-Schlatter disease, including medical professionals, coaches, educators, and parents, is one strategy to support those who have the illness.

This can assist in clearing up misunderstandings and encouraging early diagnosis and effective treatment of the illness.

Furthermore, promoting more financing and resources for Osgood-Schlatter disease research can enhance our knowledge of the illness and its available treatments.

This could entail pushing for legislative reforms that would give financing for musculoskeletal disorders top priority, supporting research projects, and taking part in fundraising campaigns.

Supporting patient advocacy groups and advocacy organizations for Osgood-Schlatter disease can also be a great way to spread the word and rally support for the condition.

These groups frequently offer tools, networks of support, and chances for advocacy to people with the illness and their families.

Individuals can significantly improve the lives of persons impacted by Osgood-Schlatter disease and support constructive change in the healthcare system and the larger community by taking part in advocacy and awareness campaigns.

CHAPTER SEVEN

RECTIFICATION METHOD

To manage Osgood-Schlatter disease (OSD), rehabilitation is essential. Its goals include symptom relief, strength restoration, and a safe transition back to physical activity. Rest, physical activity, and a gradual return to sports or other physical pursuits are usually part of the process.

Gradual Resumption Of Physical Activity

Physical activities can be progressively resumed by individuals with OSD after a period of rest to allow the damaged area to heal. To prevent aggravating symptoms, it's crucial to begin cautiously and increase duration and intensity gradually. Before moving on to more demanding sports or workouts, start with low-impact activities like cycling or swimming that don't put undue strain on your knees.

Keeping an eye on the symptoms and development

It is essential to keep a close eye on progress and symptoms over the entire rehabilitation procedure. A worsening of discomfort or swelling during or after an activity may be a sign that the knee is not prepared for that degree of activity. On the other hand, if symptoms subside with rest and suitable activity, this indicates that the rehabilitation is going well.

Sports Medicine Specialists And Physical Therapists' Roles

Sports medicine experts and physical therapists are essential in helping people with OSD navigate the recovery process. They can offer individualized treatment programs, suggest suitable exercise regimens, and give guidance on how to avoid being hurt again. To guarantee the best possible recovery, these experts regularly keep an eye on developments and modify the rehabilitation program as necessary.

Combining Fitness and Strengthening Programs

Programs for fitness and strengthening are crucial parts of OSD recovery. To improve stability and support, these programs concentrate on increasing the strength, flexibility, and endurance of the muscles that surround the knee joint.

Leg raises, squats, lunges, and core-building exercises are a few possible workouts. Stretching exercises can also aid in reducing stiffness and increasing flexibility in the surrounding muscles and knee.

Extended-Term Management Approaches

Effective symptom management and long-term recurrence prevention are equally important components of managing open-source dementia (OSD). Short-term rehabilitation is not enough. This may entail carrying out conditioning and strengthening workouts into the post-symptom phase to preserve joint stability and muscle strength. People who have OSD should also be careful about how active they are and try not to put too much or too often stress on their knees. Healthcare practitioners can detect early indicators of recurrence and take appropriate action by conducting routine monitoring.

CHAPTER EIGHT

LIFESTYLE MODIFICATIONS

Nutritional Aspects Of Healing And Recuperation

When dealing with Osgood-Schlatter disease, paying attention to your nutrition can considerably benefit the healing process. In addition to promoting bone health, a diet high in protein, calcium, and vitamin D can hasten healing. The nutrients required to support bone growth and repair can be found in foods including dairy products, leafy greens, fortified cereals, and lean meats.

A balanced diet can also aid in controlling inflammation and lessening pain related to Osgood-Schlatter disease. Anti-inflammatory foods include nuts, seeds, fatty fish, and antioxidant-rich fruits. They can also help reduce pain and accelerate healing. In addition to lowering inflammation, avoiding processed foods, sugary snacks, and too much coffee can also improve general health.

Maintaining hydration is crucial for both healing and recuperation. Maintaining optimal hydration levels in the body, lubricating joints, and eliminating toxins can all be achieved by consuming a sufficient amount of water throughout the day. Selecting natural fruit juices or water instead of sugar-filled drinks will help you stay hydrated and avoid consuming extra calories.

Ergonomic Modifications For Everyday Tasks

Adapting your daily routine to be more ergonomic can help relieve knee strain and lessen pain related to Osgood-Schlatter disease. Adjusting workstation heights to maintain a neutral posture, utilizing supportive footwear, and utilizing ergonomic chairs with enough lumbar support are just a few simple adjustments that can greatly lessen knee pain and improve alignment.

Stretching and moving around frequently after lengthy sitting or standing activities helps prevent stiffness and relieve pressure on the knees. When kneeling or sitting for prolonged amounts of time, using ergonomic items like knee pads or cushions can offer extra support and padding to lessen discomfort.

To prevent undue pressure on the knees, it's also critical to lift or carry large objects with appropriate body mechanics. Osgood-Schlatter disease symptoms can be avoided by using safe lifting practices, such as bending at the knees rather than the waist and spreading weight evenly.

Including Low-Impact Activities

While high-intensity exercise may aggravate Osgood-Schlatter disease symptoms, low-impact exercise might assist preserve mobility, flexibility, and strength without exacerbating knee discomfort. For those with Osgood-Schlatter disease, walking, cycling, and swimming are great options because they improve cardiovascular health without placing undue strain on the knees.

Additionally helpful for enhancing flexibility and balance as well as strengthening the muscles around the knees are yoga and pilates. To prevent overexertion, it's crucial to stay away from poses or exercises that worsen knee pain and to pay attention to your body's cues.

Regular mobility and stretching exercises can help relieve Osgood-Schlatter disease-related joint stiffness and enhance joint function. To keep your knees flexible and within range of motion, concentrate on doing light stretches that work your quadriceps, hamstrings, and calves.

The Value Of Getting Enough Sleep And Rest

The body can recover from Osgood-Schlatter disease by repairing damaged tissues and reducing inflammation, which is made possible by rest and sleep. Prioritizing enough rest and sleep is crucial for accelerating healing and avoiding symptom aggravation.

Aim for seven to nine hours of unbroken sleep each night to ensure you're getting enough sleep to let your body recover and rejuvenate. Establishing a soothing evening routine that includes deep breathing exercises, a warm bath, or soothing music might help improve the quality of sleep and speed up the healing process.

Including rest intervals during the day, in addition to sleeping at night, can help avoid overuse problems and lessen knee strain. To avoid making your Osgood-Schlatter disease symptoms worse, pay attention to your body's cues and take breaks when necessary when engaging in physical activity or spending extended amounts of time standing or sitting still.

Taking Rest Periods And Physical Activity Into Account

Maintaining Osgood-Schlatter disease and avoiding overuse injuries requires striking the correct balance between exercise and rest times. While having an active lifestyle is crucial for general health and well-being, it's also critical to give yourself enough time to relax and recover to avoid aggravating existing conditions.

To give your body time to heal and mend, think about including rest days or low-impact activities in your exercise regimen. Low-impact exercises and high-intensity workouts alternately can help minimize knee strain and prevent overuse issues.

Pay attention to the cues your body gives you and modify the amount of activity you do. Reduce the amount of time or intensity of your physical activity if you feel more pain or discomfort during or after it to prevent aggravating your symptoms. Recall that to support healing and recovery from Osgood-Schlatter disease, rest is equally as crucial as activity.

CHAPTER NINE

RESEARCH DIRECTIONS AND FUTURE STEPS

New Approaches To Treatment

There is promise for better management of Osgood Schlatter Disease (OSD) as novel therapeutic options for the ailment continue to emerge as medical research develops. Non-invasive therapies that seek to reduce pain and accelerate recovery without requiring surgery represent one promising area of development. These techniques frequently target correcting biomechanical alignment, strengthening the afflicted muscles and tendons, and lowering inflammation.

Using regenerative medicine procedures like stem cell injections and platelet-rich plasma (PRP) therapy is one new treatment modality that is gaining popularity. To promote tissue healing and regeneration, PRP therapy entails injecting a concentrated solution of the patient's platelets into the injured area. Similar to this, stem cell injections try to use the body's healing processes by infusing stem cells into the injured area, which may hasten recovery and lessen discomfort.

Using innovative rehabilitation procedures designed especially for people with OSD is another viable strategy. To increase muscle strength, flexibility, and general function, these programs may combine stretches, exercises, and physical therapy methods. Through the treatment of underlying muscular imbalances and biomechanical problems, these programs aim to improve functional results and lessen pain in people with OSD.

Researchers are looking into the possible advantages of complementary and alternative medicine practices including acupuncture, chiropractic adjustments, and herbal supplements in addition to these cutting-edge treatments. Although more investigation is required to evaluate these methods' effectiveness in treating OSD, they show potential as complementary therapies that could aid afflicted people's quality of life and reduce symptoms.

Progress In Diagnostic Methods

Osgood Schlatter Disease (OSD) must be diagnosed accurately to be effectively managed, and new developments in diagnostic methods have improved our capacity to recognize and evaluate the illness more precisely. Conventional diagnostic techniques, such as physical examinations and reviews of medical histories, are still vital steps in the diagnosis process because they enable medical professionals to analyze symptoms, determine risk factors, and rule out other explanations for knee pain.

However, improvements in imaging technologies have completely changed how OSD is diagnosed and given doctors important new knowledge about the underlying anatomical abnormalities that underlie the illness. Accurate evaluation of the tendon inflammation, fragmentation, and ossification typical of OSD is made possible by the thorough view of the patellar tendon and adjacent tissues provided by magnetic resonance imaging (MRI) and ultrasound imaging modalities.

Furthermore, real-time imaging of the knee joint during dynamic motions is now possible because of improvements in musculoskeletal ultrasound technology, which makes it possible to monitor patellar tendon function and biomechanics dynamically. When assessing functional deficits and determining contributing factors such as aberrant patellar tracking or weakness in the quadriceps muscle, this dynamic imaging capacity is especially helpful.

Emerging diagnostic techniques including ultrasonic biomicroscopy (UBM) and shear wave elastography (SWE), in addition to conventional imaging modalities, show promise for evaluating tissue stiffness and microstructural alterations linked to OSD. Quantitative assessments of tendon elasticity and morphology are made possible by these non-invasive procedures, which enable the early detection of tendon pathology and the long-term monitoring of therapy response.

Through the implementation of these sophisticated diagnostic methods in clinical settings, medical professionals may enhance the precision of OSD diagnosis, customize treatment plans to meet the specific requirements of each patient, and maximize results for those afflicted with this prevalent teenage knee ailment.

Knowing The Long-Term Prognosis

Even though Osgood Schlatter Disease (OSD) usually gets better with time and proper care, knowing the condition's long-term prognosis is crucial for directing treatment choices and setting realistic expectations for patients. Studies that follow people with a history of OSD into adulthood have yielded important insights into how the illness progresses naturally and how it might affect musculoskeletal health in later life.

A significant discovery from long-term studies is that most people with OSD benefit from conservative treatment, such as activity modification, physical therapy, and pain management techniques, which results in symptom resolution and functional improvement. Still, some people may experience lingering symptoms like infrequent knee pain or stiffness, especially if they play high-impact sports or engage in other activities that put an excessive amount of strain on their patellar tendon.

Long-term follow-up studies have also found potential risk factors, such as bilateral or severe OSD, aberrant patellar tracking, and chronic quadriceps muscle weakness, for both persistent symptoms and functional difficulties in adulthood. People who have these risk factors may benefit from focused therapies and continuous monitoring to manage lingering symptoms and avoid chronic consequences like osteoarthritis in the knee or patellar tendinopathy.

To lower the likelihood of repeat injury and long-term musculoskeletal dysfunction, it is also critical to optimize muscular balance and biomechanical alignment during adolescence, according to a recent study. Optimizing musculoskeletal health throughout life may be facilitated by interventions that enhance lower extremity strength, flexibility, and neuromuscular control. These measures may also help lessen the long-term effects of osteoarthritis.

Healthcare professionals can create customized treatment plans that address both immediate symptom relief and long-term musculoskeletal health for patients affected by this common adolescent knee condition by learning more about the long-term prognosis of OSD and identifying factors that influence outcomes.

www.ingramcontent.com/pod-product-compliance
Lightning Source LLC
Chambersburg PA
CBHW071840210526
45479CB00001B/221